KB & NASH

Written by

JoBeth Souza · Elizabeth Olear · Karabeth Souza

Illustrated by Ahmad Sabadunya

ISBN: 979-8-9904197-1-1

Illustrated by Ahmad Sabadunya

Produced by Publish Pros | publishpros.com

Dedication

JoBeth: To Jax and Em for being the best elementary school friends KB could have. To my parents for your love, support, encouragement, assistance, and monetary donations throughout the years. To Evan, your science mind has always been a great resource for our family. Thank you for being the best big brother to KB. To Susan, Shannon, and The XLH Network for being a resource I found the day KB was diagnosed with XLH. It was life changing for us to find our community and not to feel like we were stranded alone on an island. Thank you for being there for us and so many other XLHers.

Elizabeth: For all children with XLH, especially those who have passed through the doors of the Yale Center for XLH.

Karabeth: I dedicate this book to my brother, Evan, who always puts me first. Thank you for all you do. I love you.

Karen Elizabeth was a very special little girl.
Her friends and family called her KB.
Her nickname was not the only thing
about KB that was short.

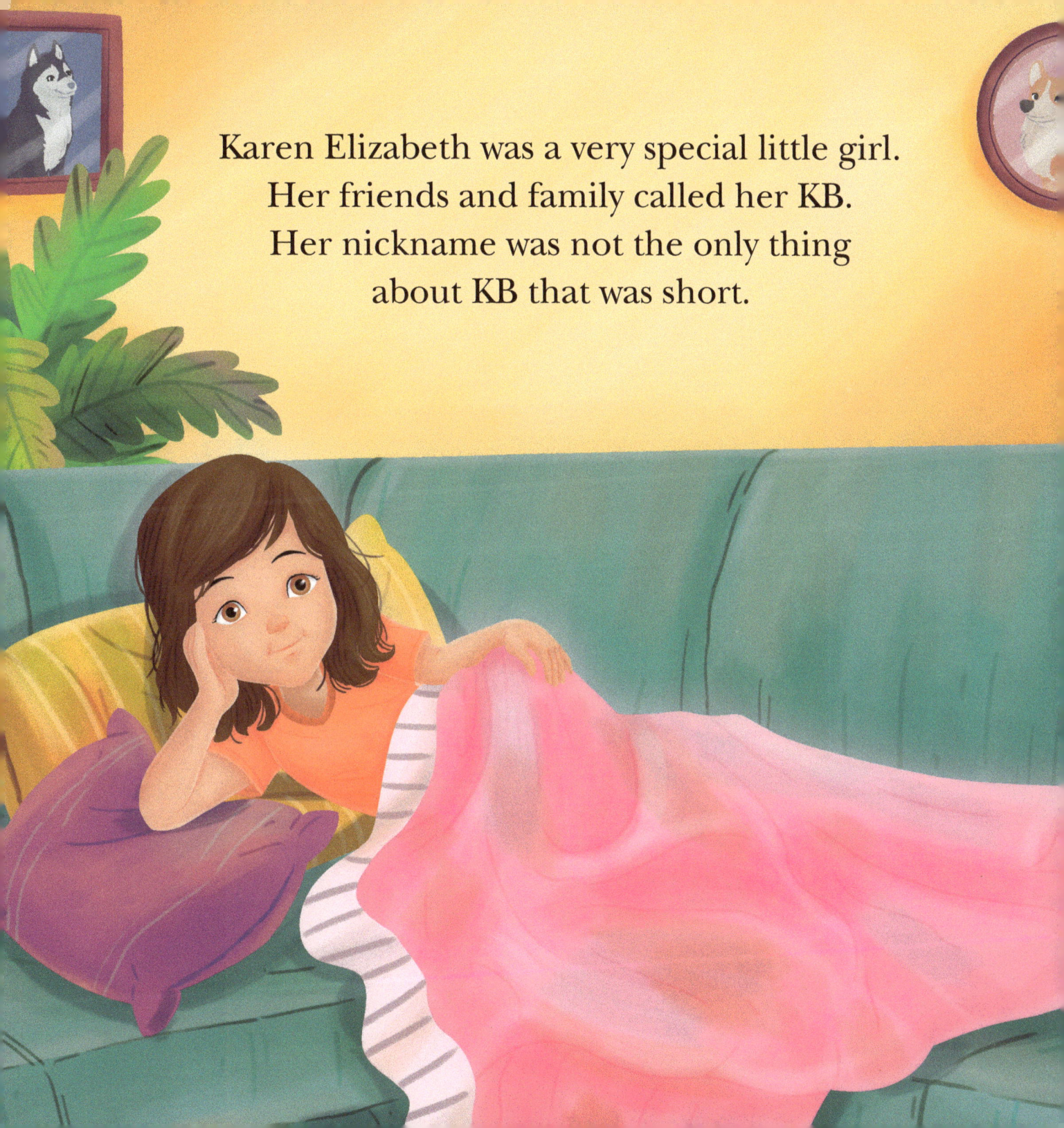

KB was shorter than other kids her age.

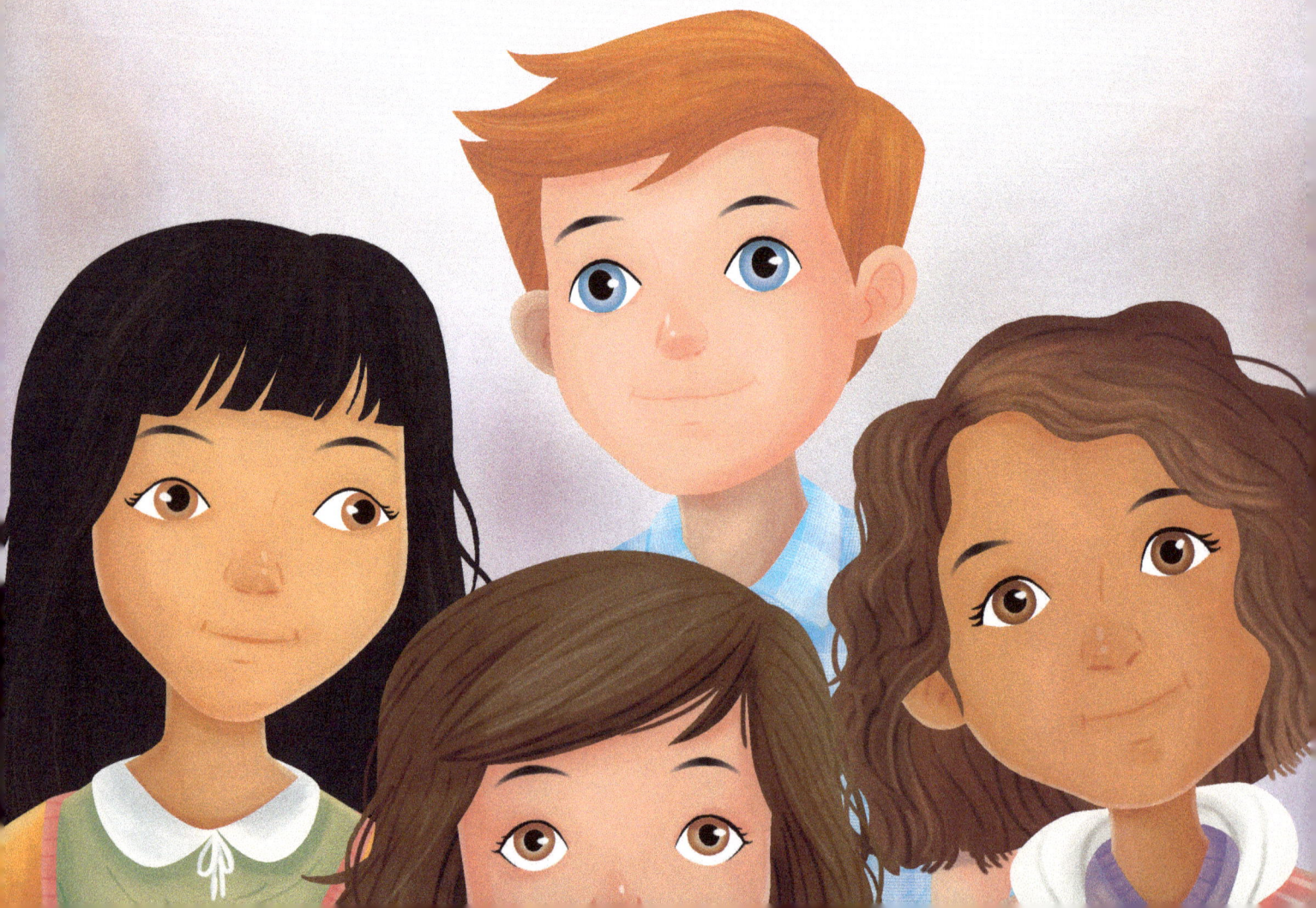

Her legs were curved,
and she wore clunky
braces until she was four.

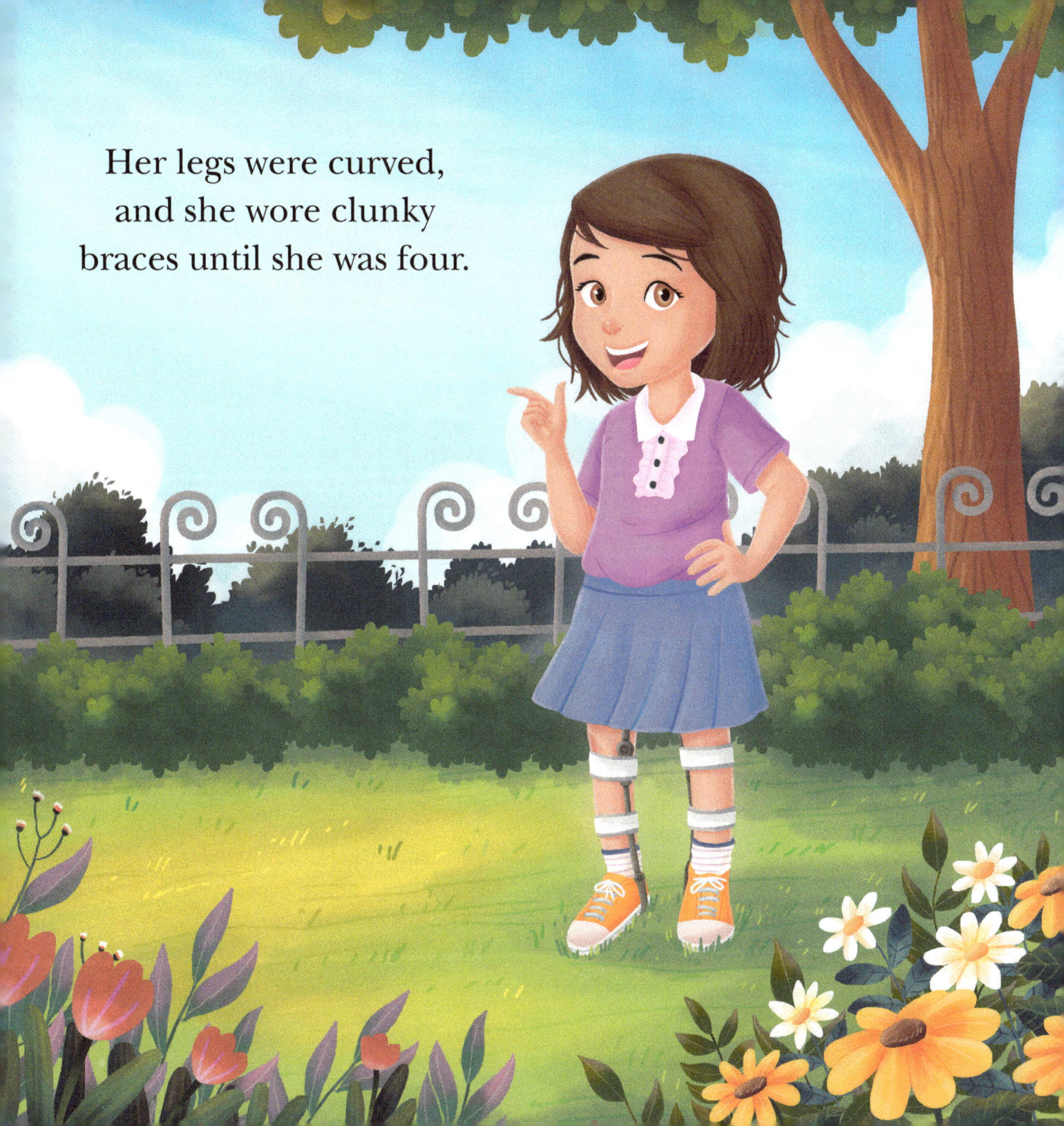

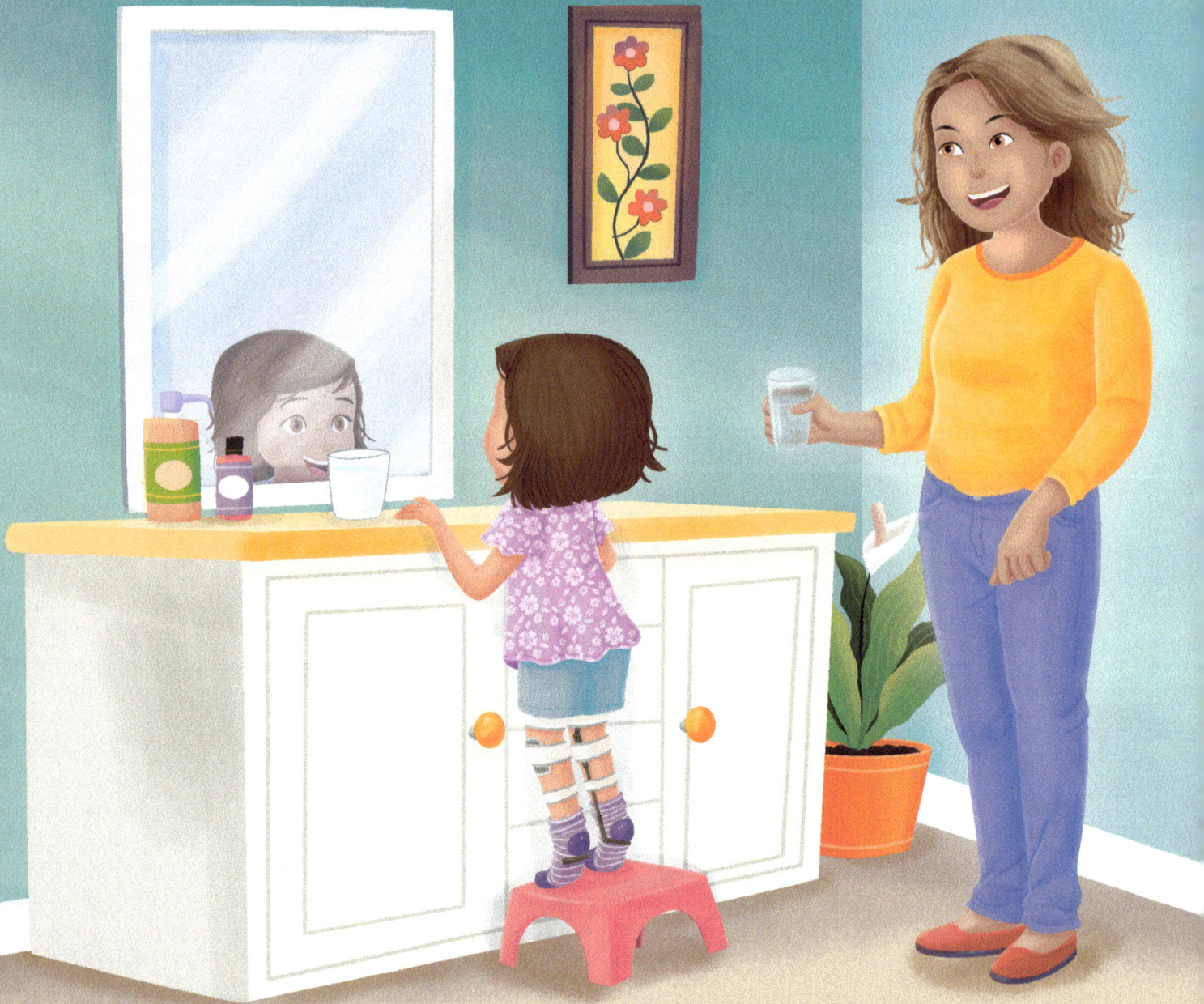

KB took medicine to help her bones grow strong.

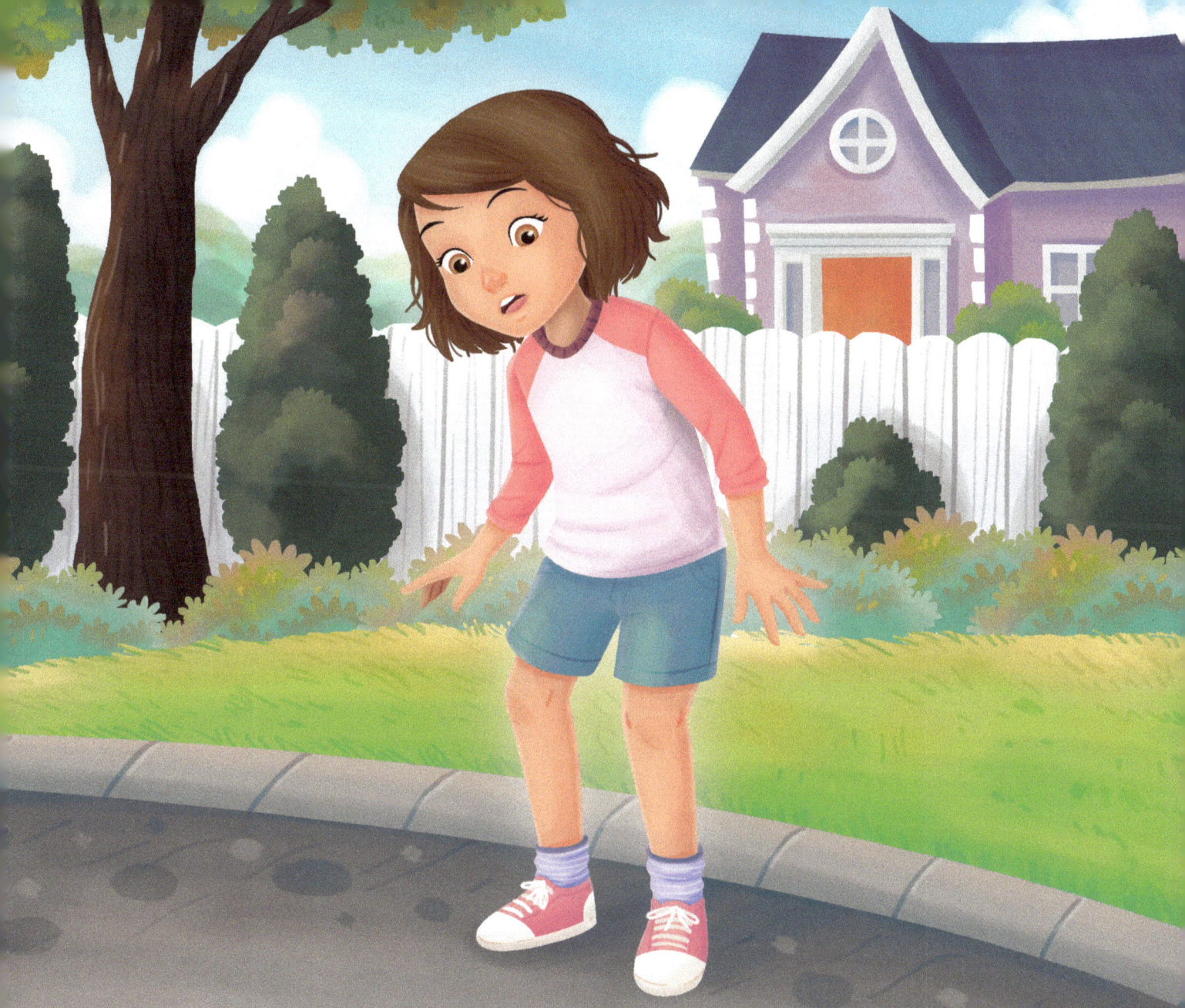

After she had surgeries to fix her legs,
she had scars on her knees.

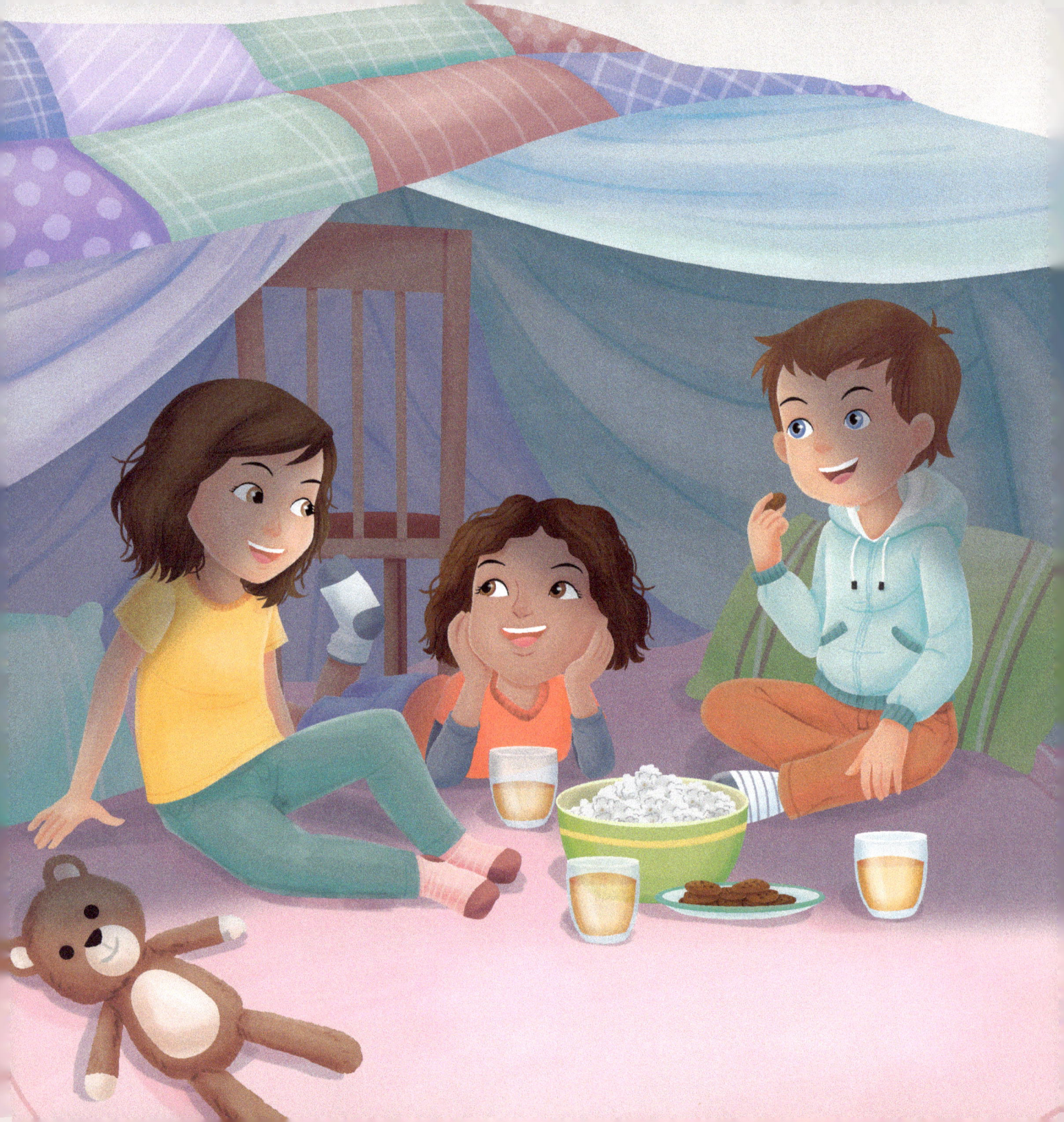

These things made KB feel different, but there were many ways she was the same as other kids her age.

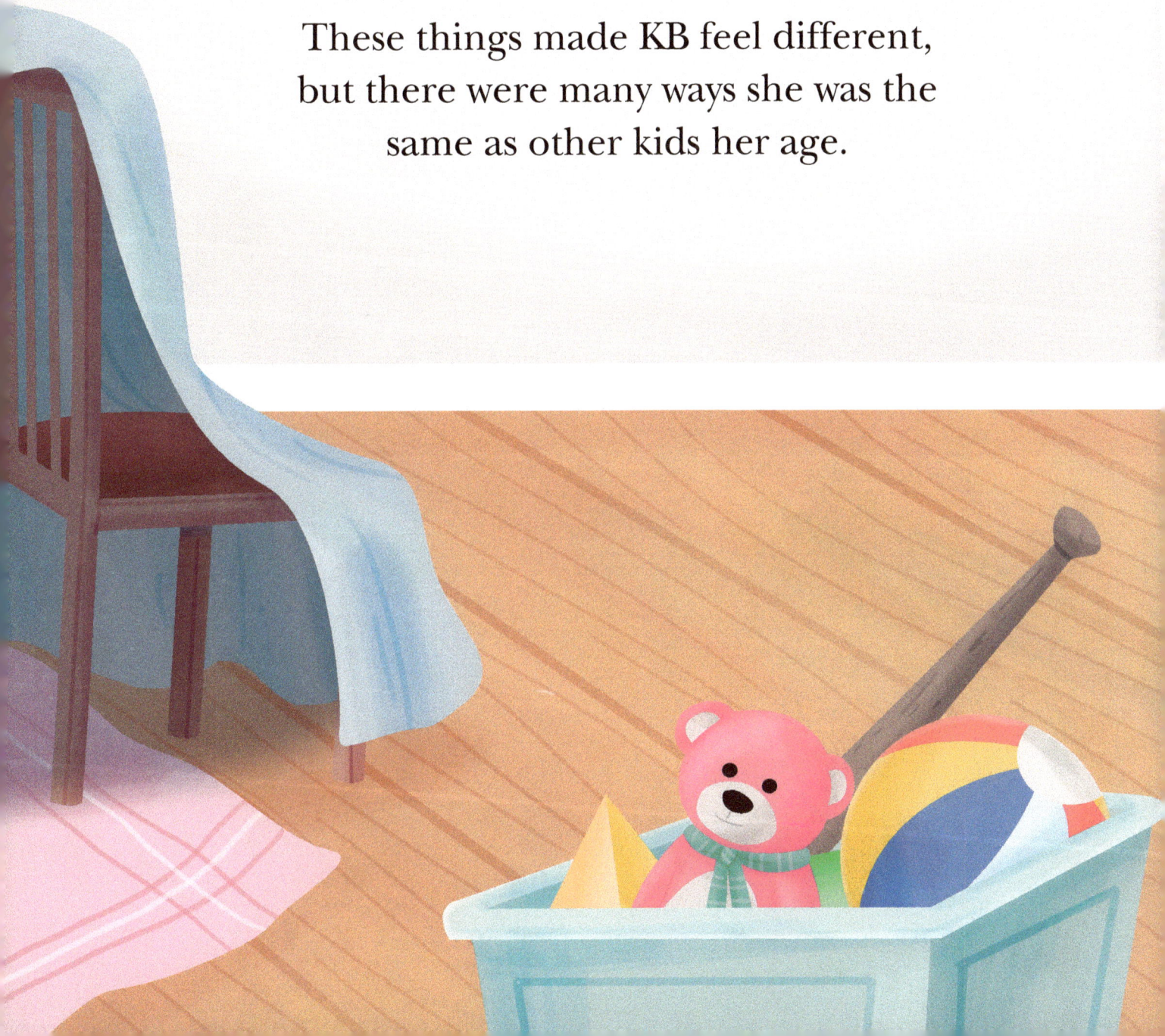

She played soccer.

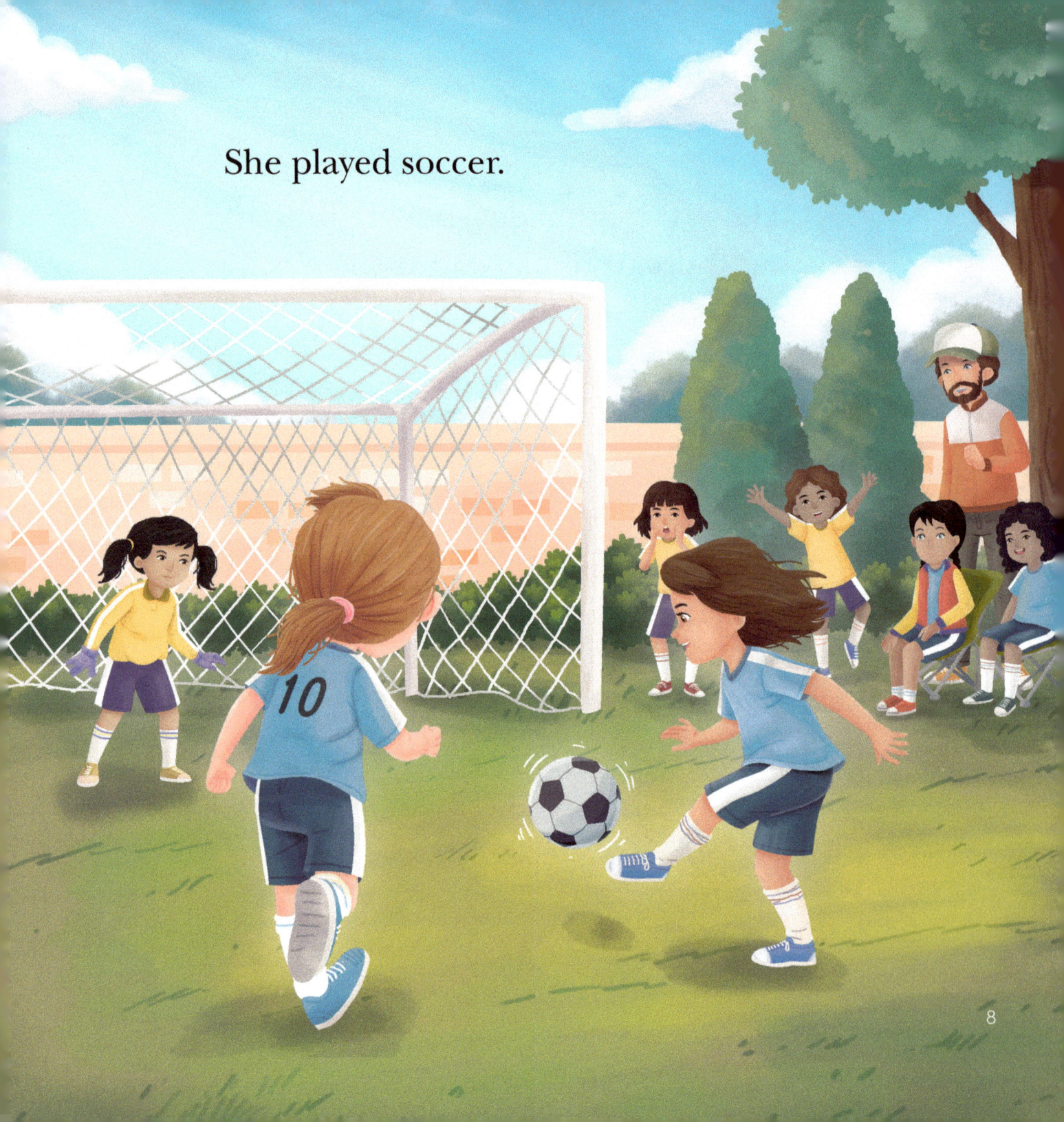

She loved music.
She took ukulele and piano lessons.

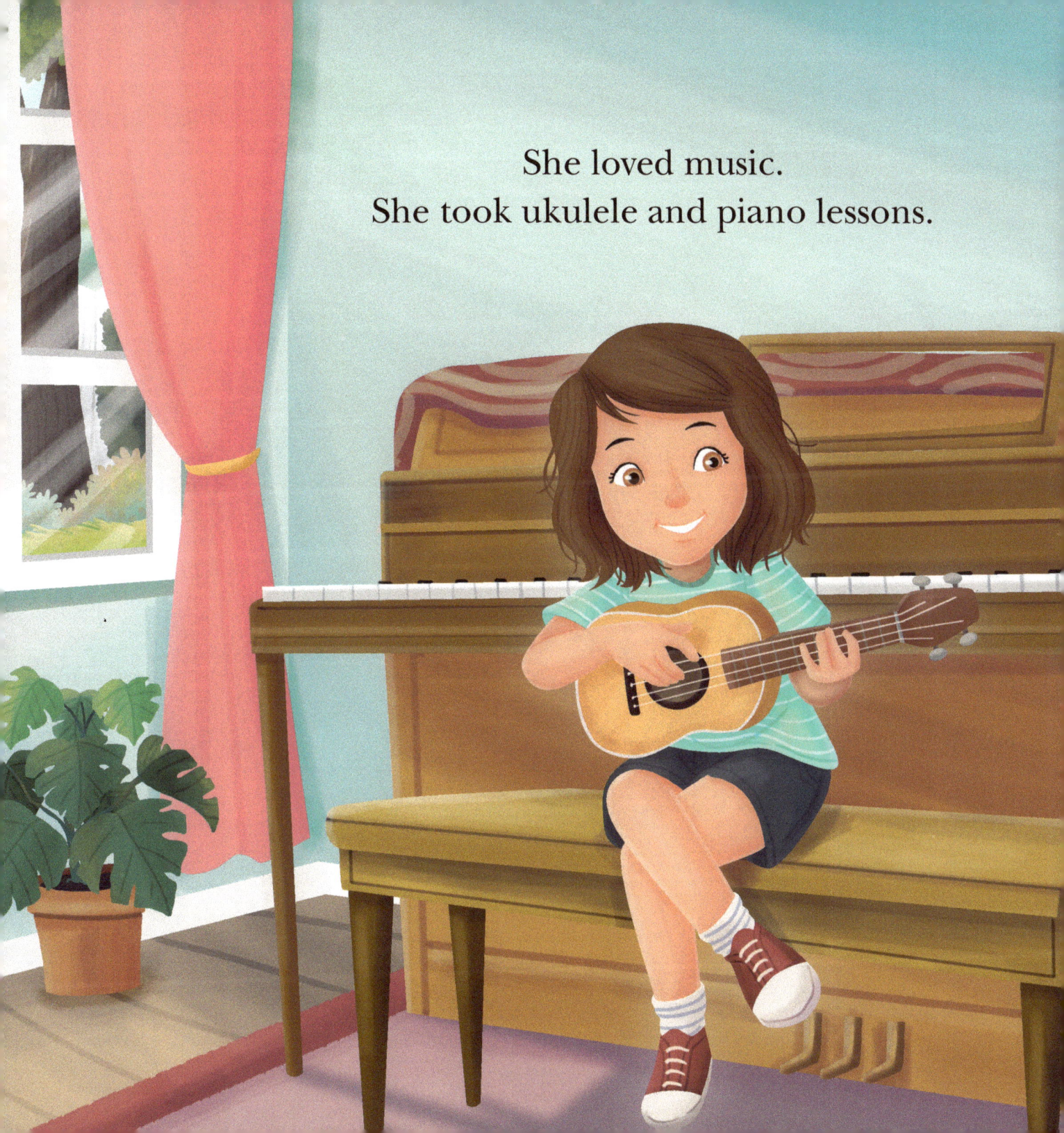

She loved dancing. She took ballet classes.

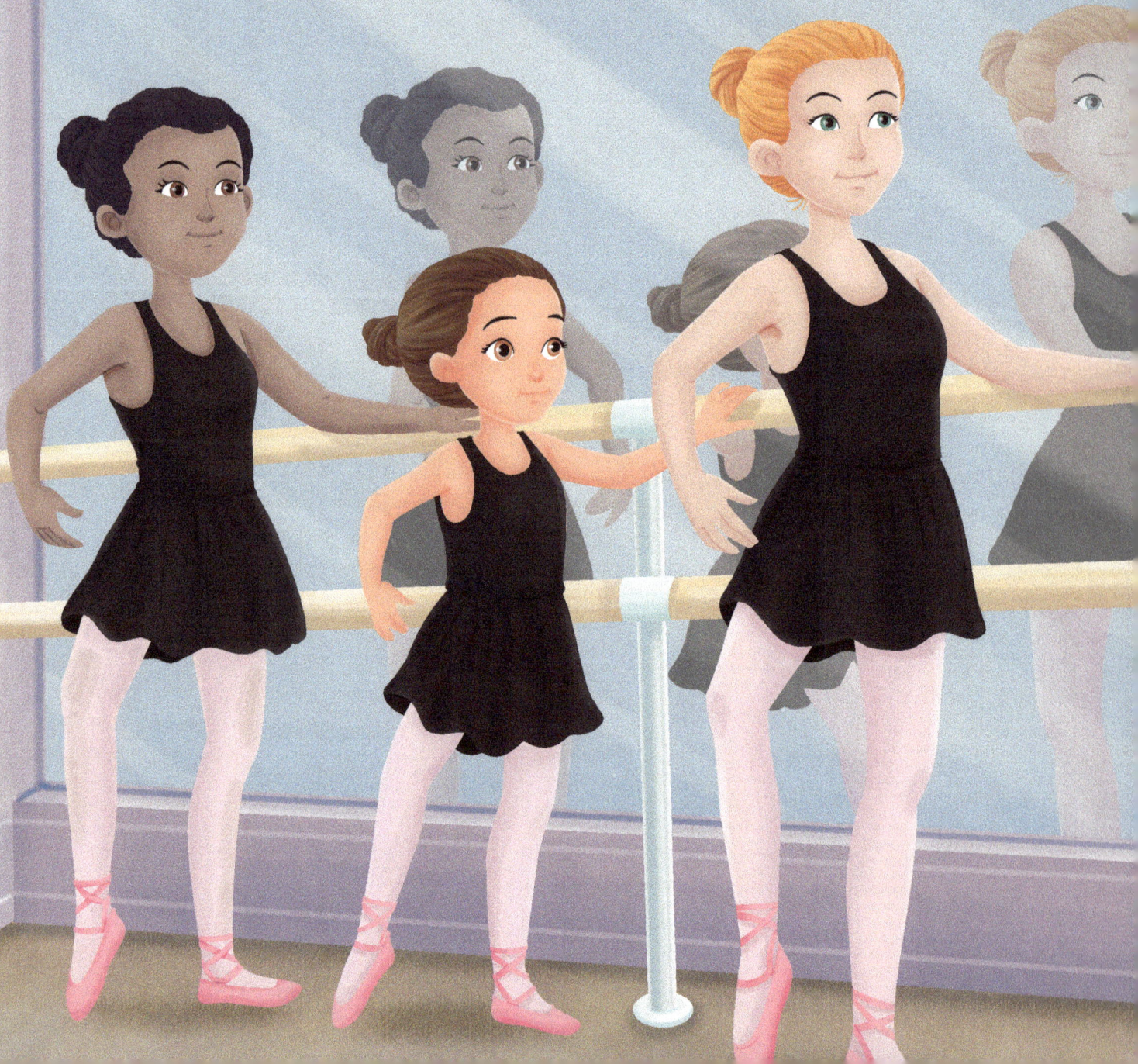

The kids at school asked why KB was short, why her legs were curved, and why she took medicine at school. The questions made KB feel sad.

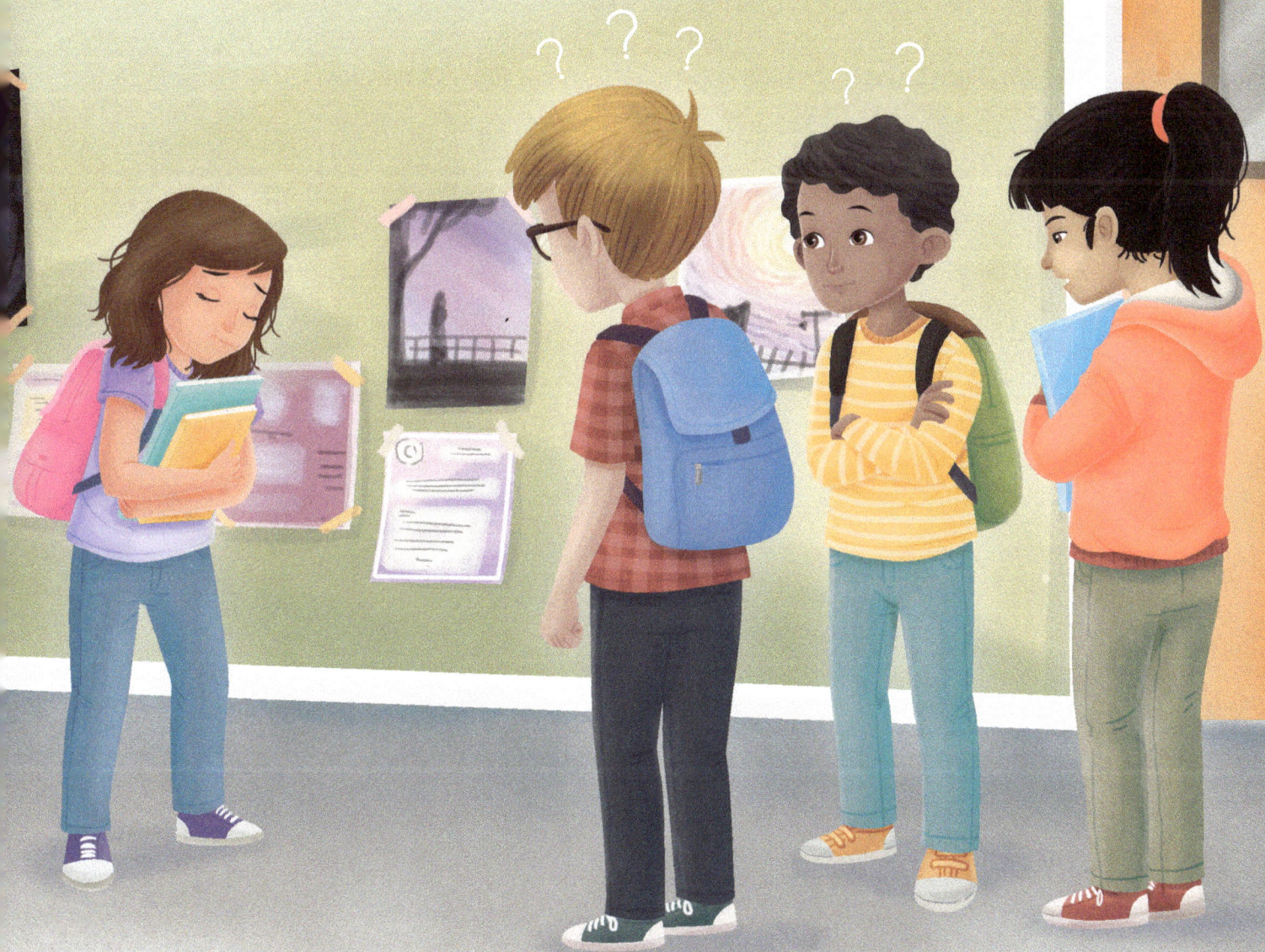

When kids asked why she had scars on her knees, KB decided to only wear pants.

She wore pants even when it was hot outside! But one day all that changed.

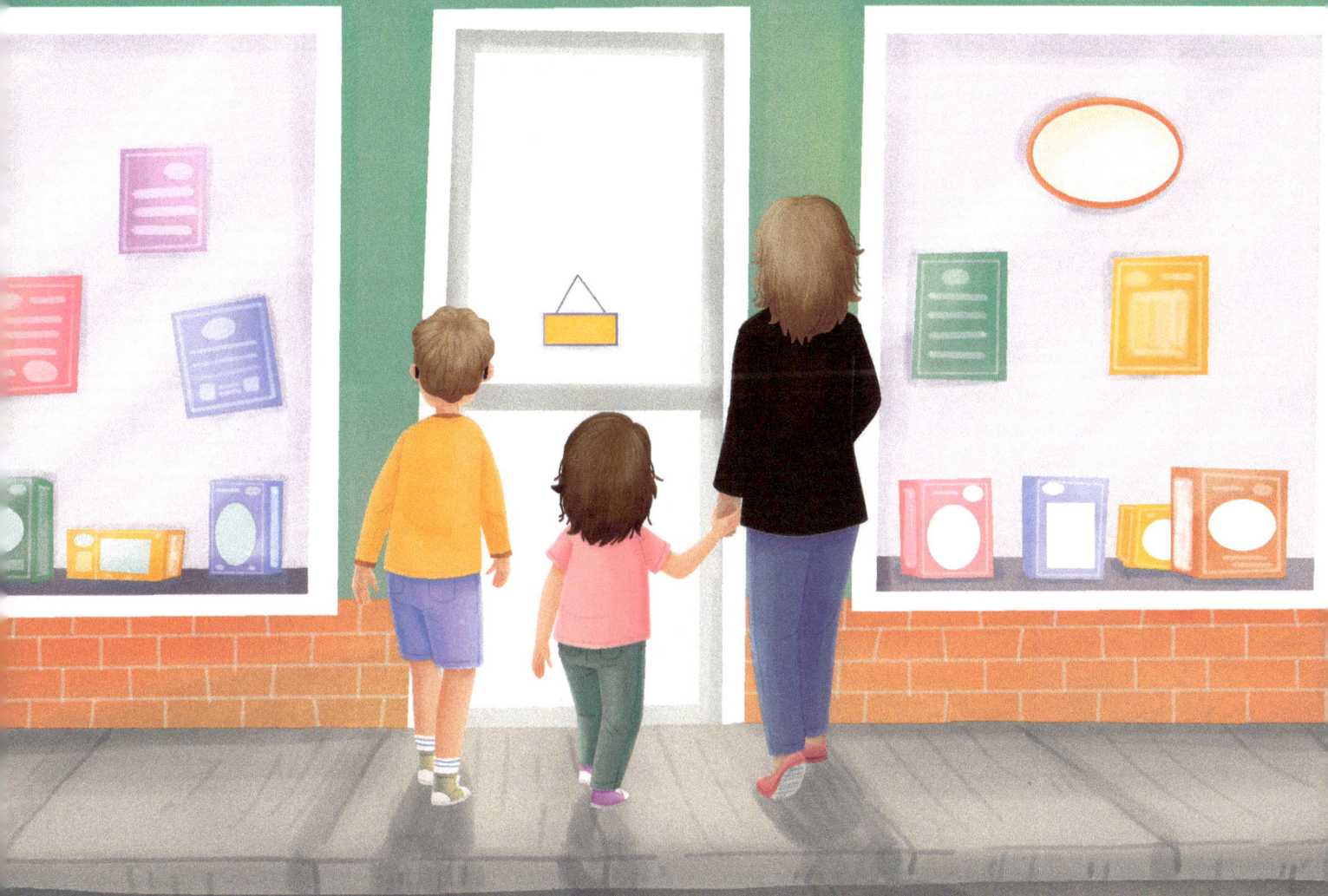

KB, her brother Evan, and her mom visited a pet store.

The pet store was having an adoption fair. KB's dad had always wanted a dog, but KB's mom thought dogs were smelly and messy.

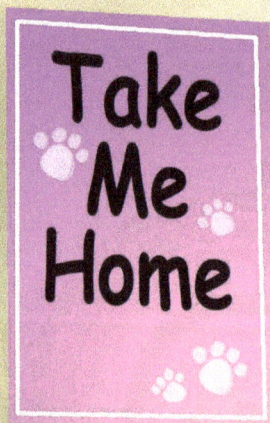

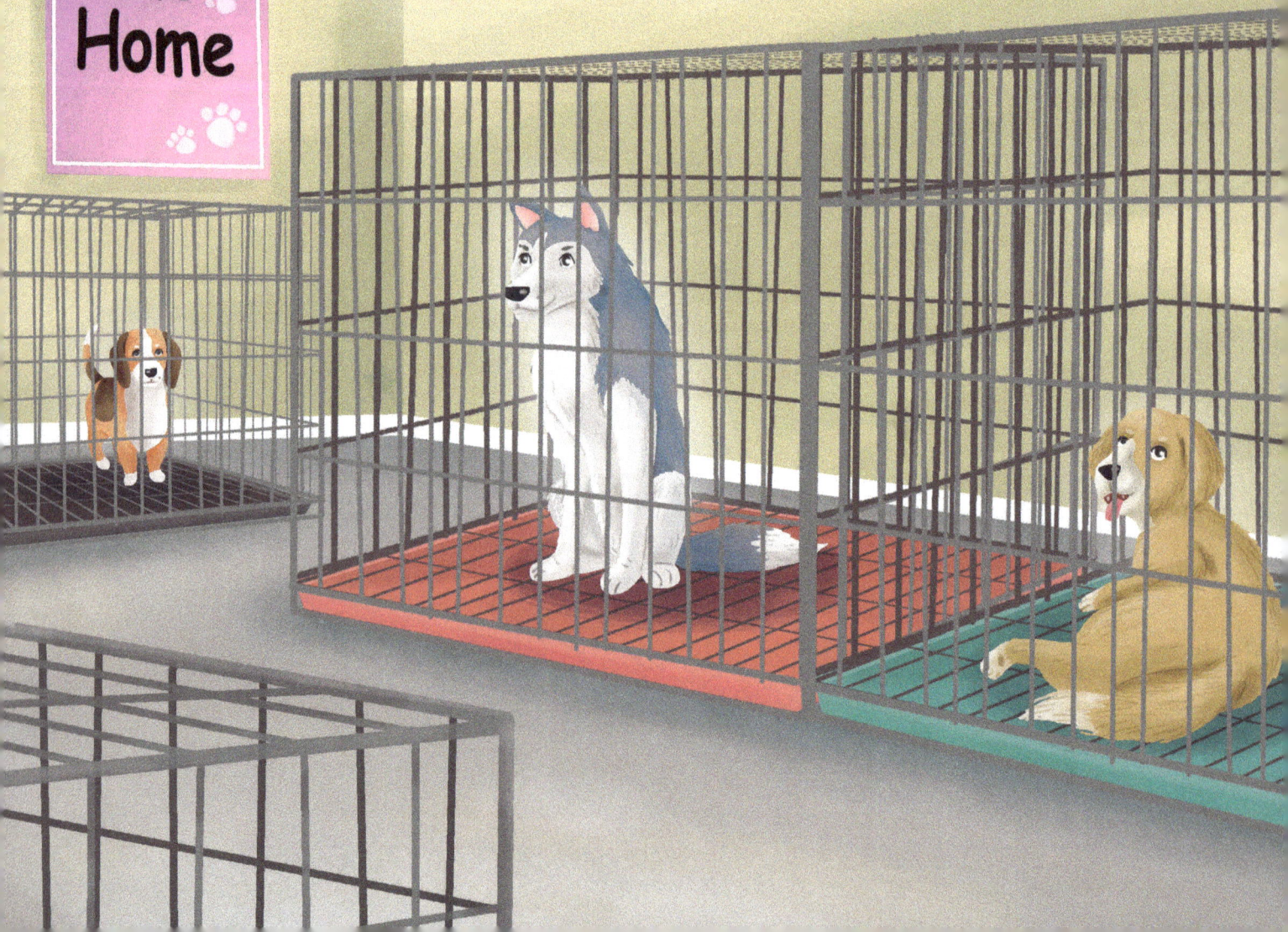

Take Me Home

ADOPT
A PET

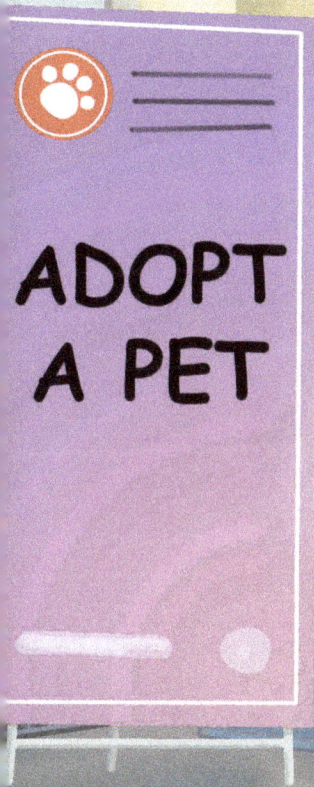

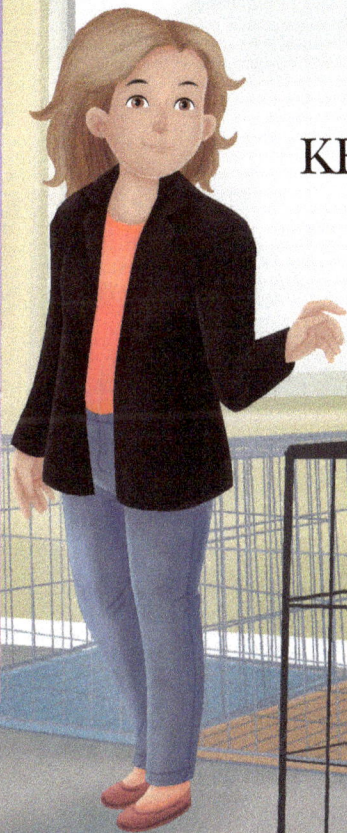

KB's mom noticed
one puppy.

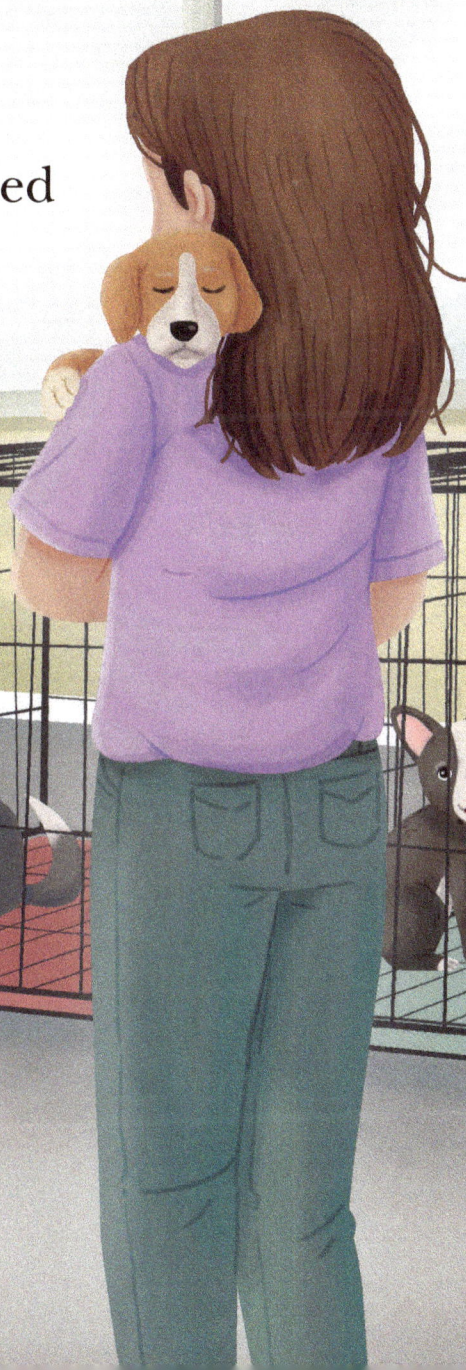

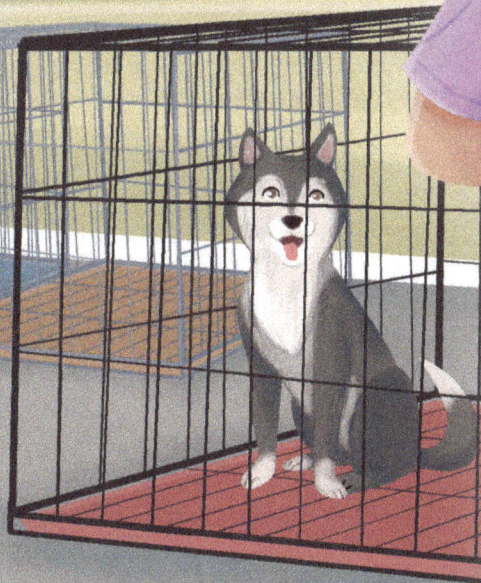

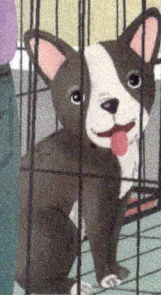

He was yellow and was fast asleep in a
worker's arms in the noisy store.

His name was Nash. The worker told
them Nash had Rickets.

KB, Evan, and their mom
could not believe their ears.

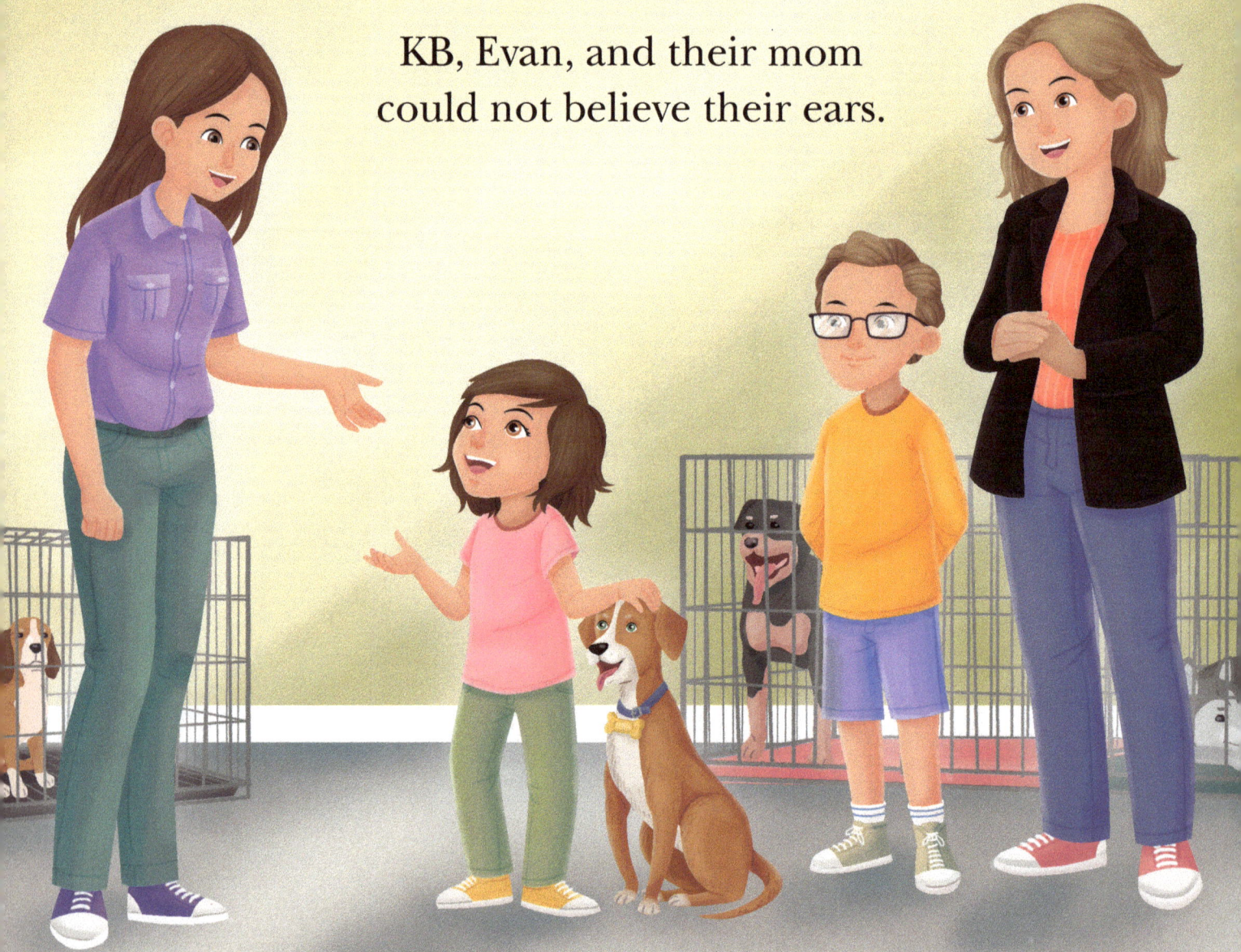

"I know what Rickets is," KB said.
"It is part of my XLH."

KB's family did not know a dog could
have Rickets. They wanted to adopt
Nash because he was special.

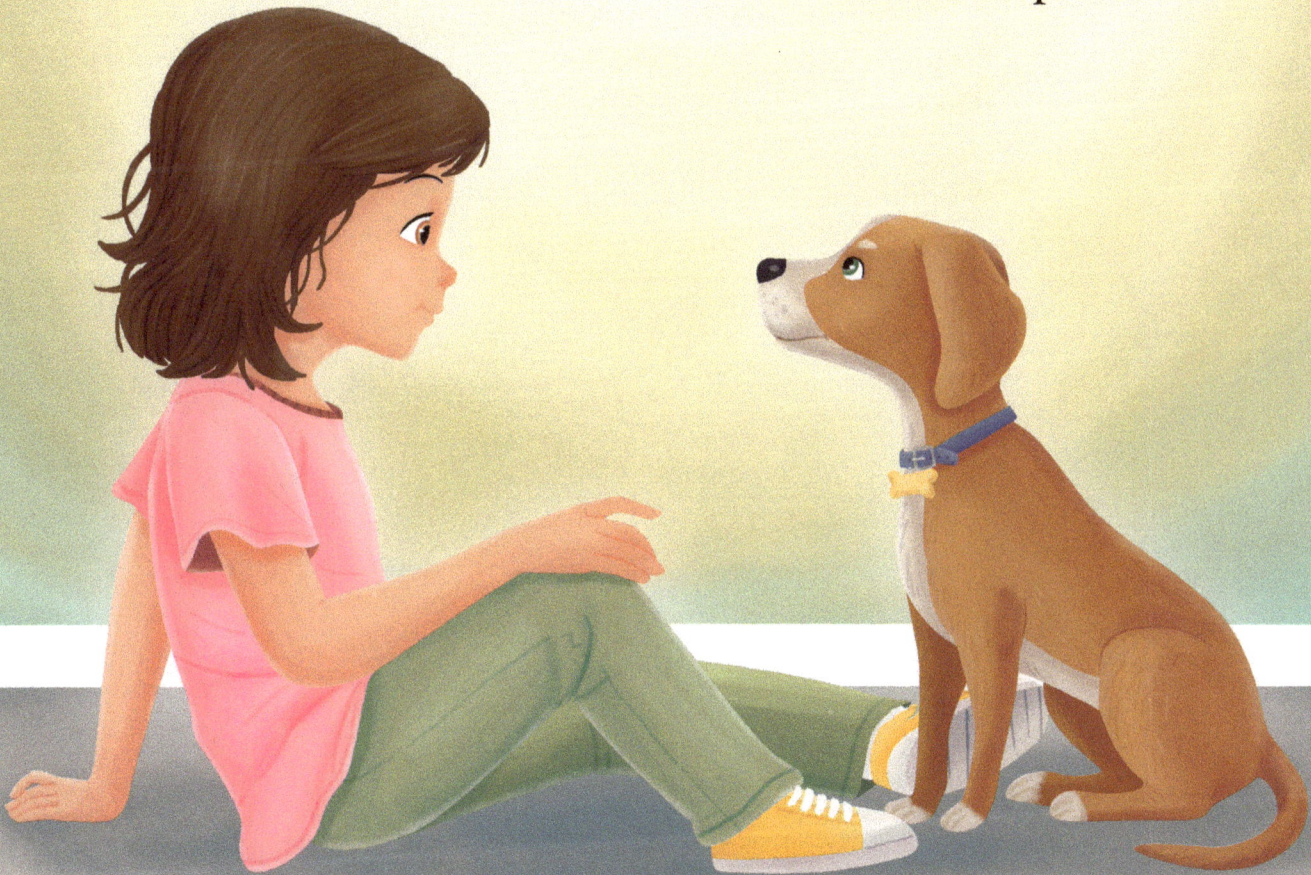

Nash was going home with them!

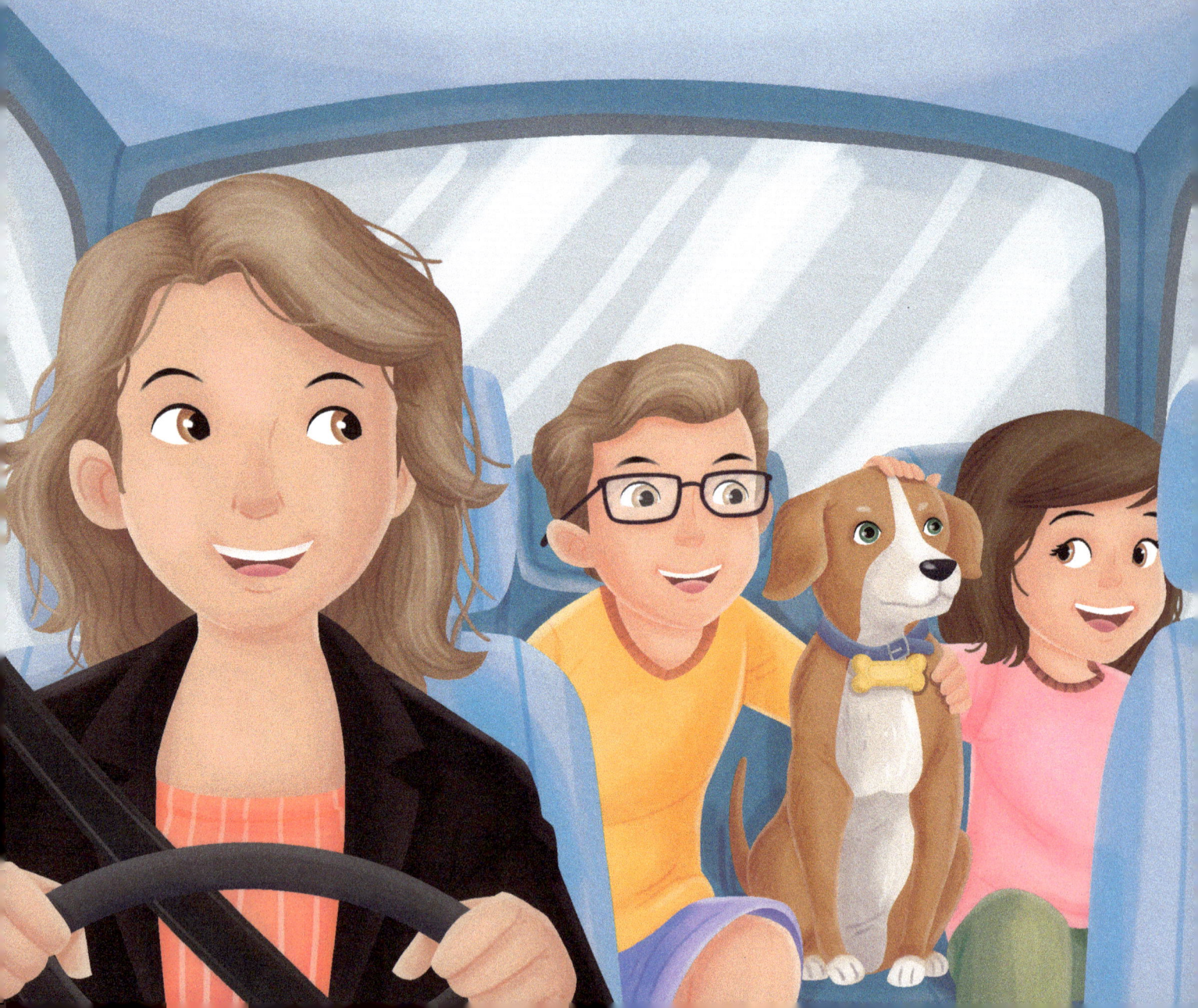

KB was so excited to have a dog just like her! They were both short, had curved legs, and had to take medicine every day to make their legs strong!

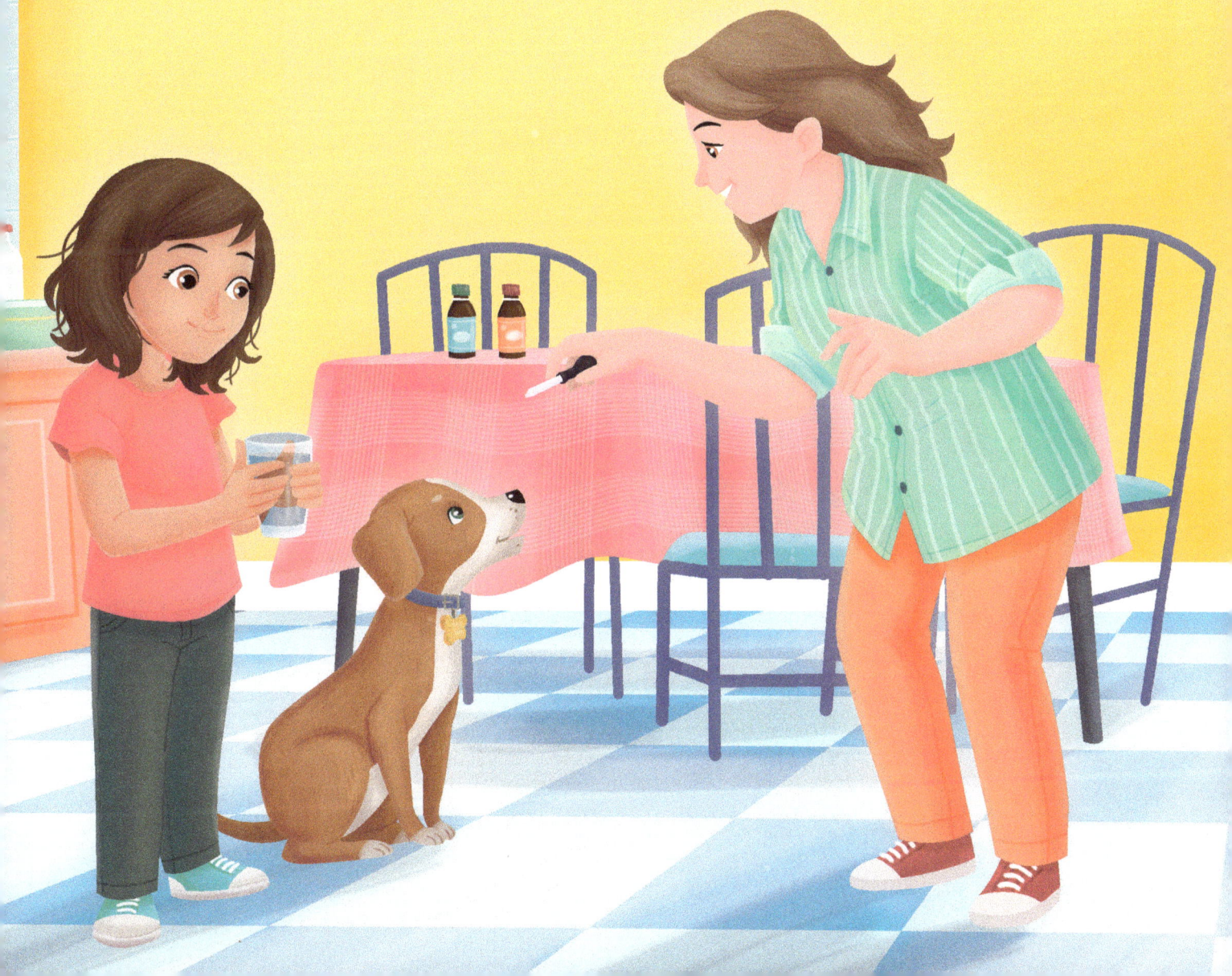

KB told everyone about her new dog, Nash. She said he was special because of his Rickets. KB started telling everyone about her XLH.

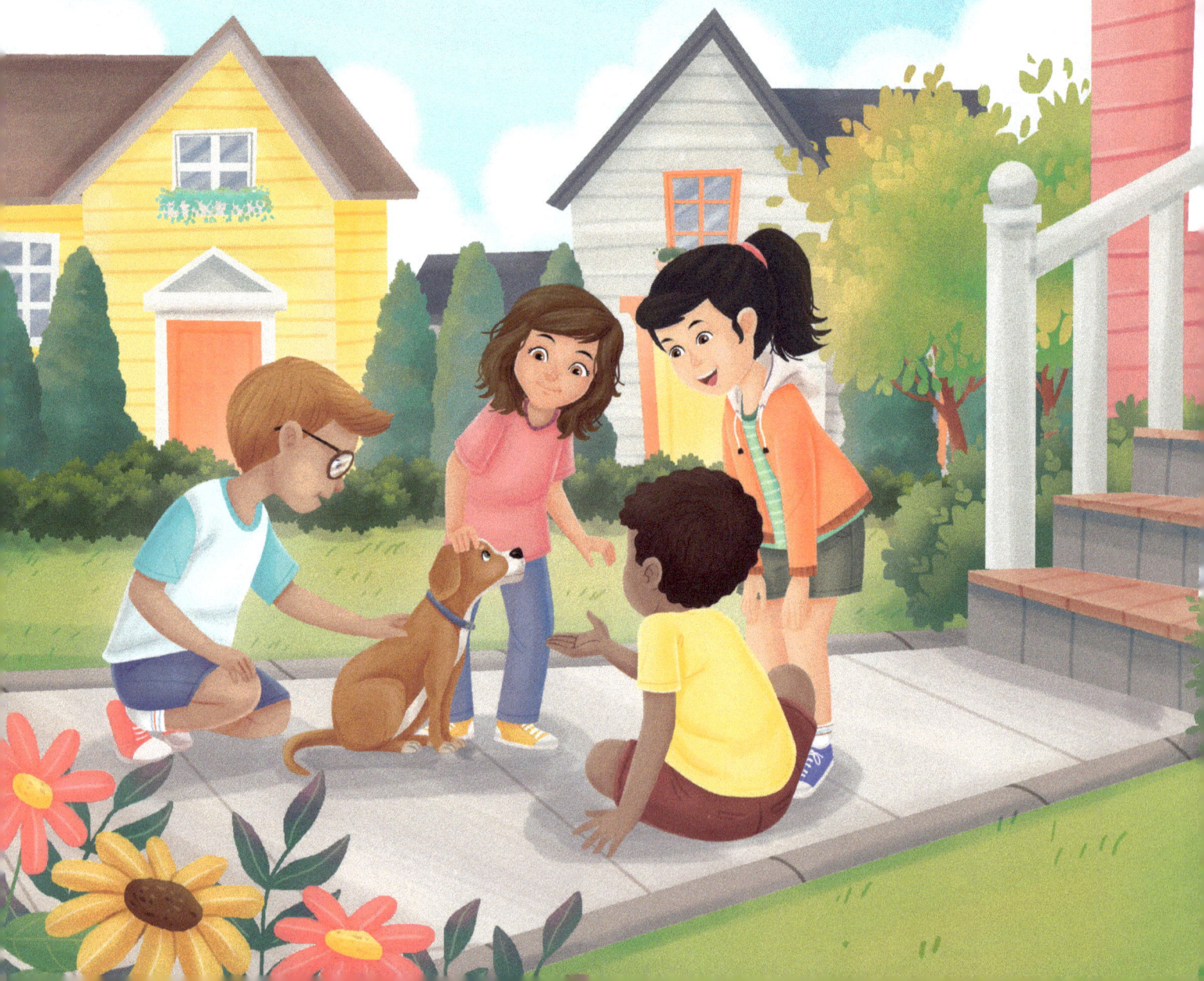

She started wearing shorts so everyone could see how Nash's legs looked like hers.

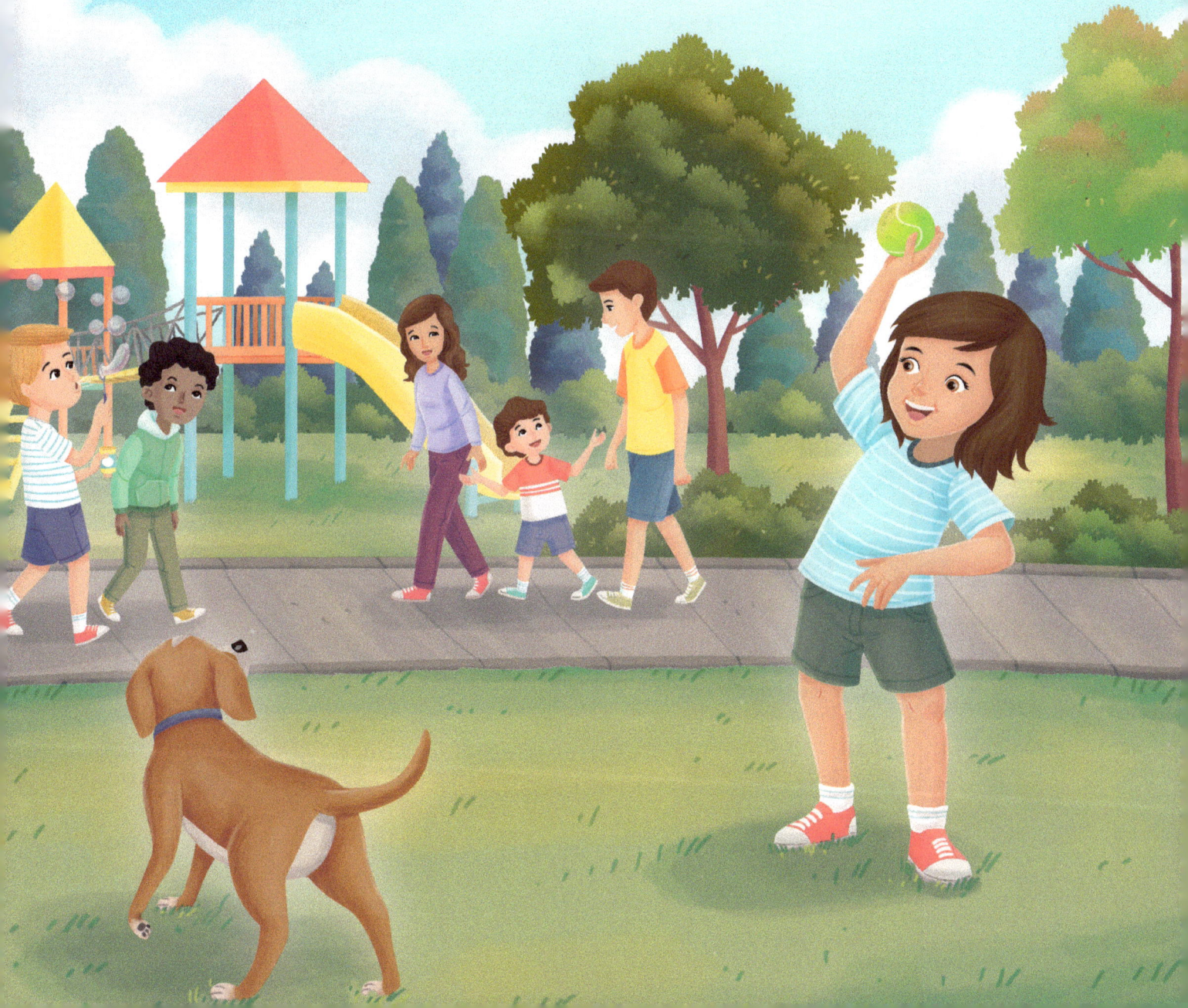

Everyone in the family loved Nash, but KB loved him most of all. And KB was Nash's favorite person.

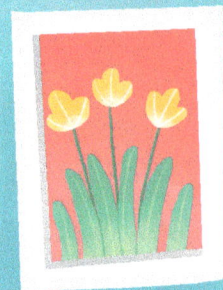

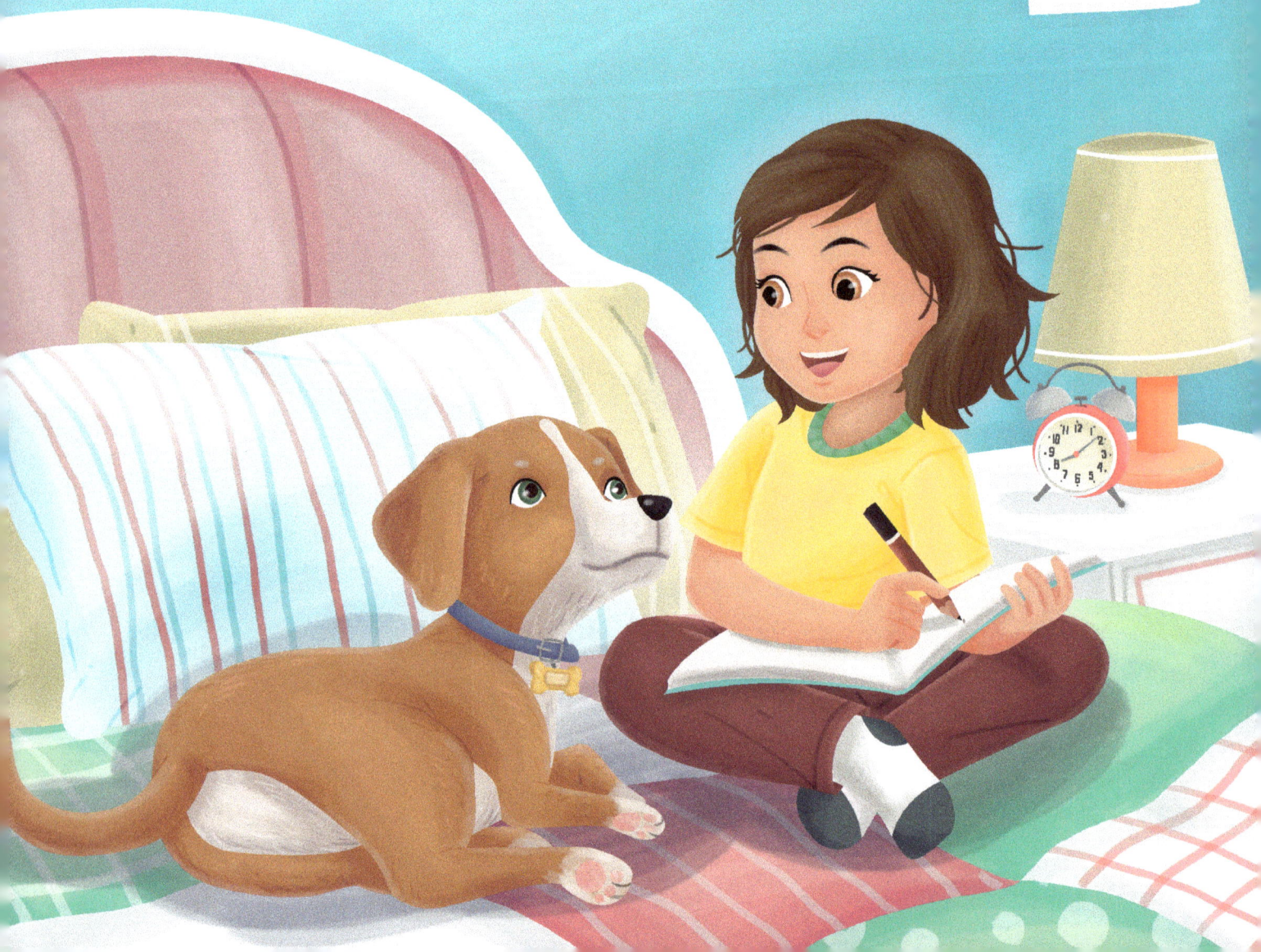

Nash helped KB realize everyone is different, and differences make people—and dogs—special.

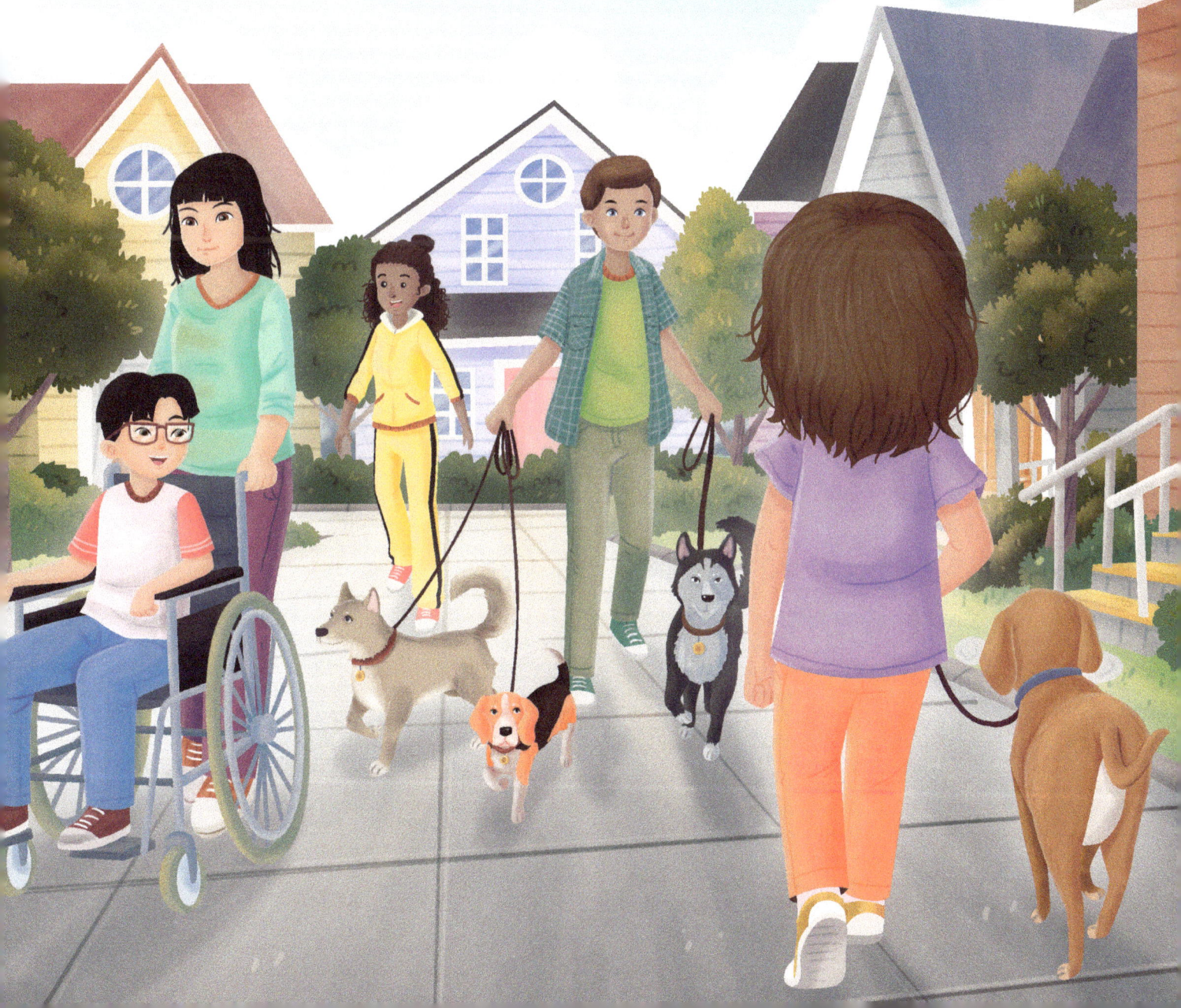

Dear Reader,

Thank you for your interest in the story of KB and Nash, and for the opportunity to share about the rare disorder of X-linked hypophosphatemia (XLH).

XLH is just one of over 10,000 rare disorders affecting more than 30 million Americans and 400 million people worldwide. This means that 1 in 10 people are living with a rare disease, and 50% of those diagnosed are children.

XLH affects 1 in 20,000 people and is characterized by low phosphorus in the blood, a consequence of a gene mutation on the X chromosome. Patients like KB experience a variety of symptoms typically related to their bones and teeth.

It is our wish that in sharing the story of KB and Nash, we bring hope to all those living with XLH or any other rare condition. You are not alone. We are all stronger together.

We hope you all find your Nash.

- JBS, EAO and KBS

For more information about XLH and other rare disorders please visit the following:

The XLH Network, Inc.: xlhnetwork.org
National Organization for Rare Disorders | NORD: rarediseases.org
Global Genes: globalgenes.org

About the Authors

JoBeth Souza, mother of KB and Evan Souza, has been passionately advocating for children with XLH since KB's diagnosis in 2008. She has played an active role in The XLH Network, serving on the board of directors and as president. She received her degree from Wake Forest University in 1992 and has worked in the securities industry since 1993. JoBeth enjoys taking piano and dance lessons, kayaking, volunteering in her community and church, and spending time with her family. She is honored to have authored this book with KB and Elizabeth.

Elizabeth Olear is the Senior Clinical Research Associate in Pediatric Endocrinology at The Yale Center for XLH. She received a Master's degree in Child Development from Tufts University, as well as a Master's in Medical Science from Boston University School of Medicine. Elizabeth is passionate about advocacy, education, and support for those with rare metabolic bone disorders and their families. She is an avid reader of books for both adults and children and enjoys traveling and sharing new recipes with her family and friends. She is honored to have co-authored this book with KB and JoBeth.

Karabeth Souza, or KB as she is known by her friends and family, was born and raised in Winston-Salem, North Carolina. Living with X Linked Hypophosphatemic Rickets (XLH) has inspired KB to raise awareness of rare childhood diseases and to volunteer with The XLH Network. She would like to major in sports medicine. KB enjoys traveling, watching and playing sports, and hanging out with her friends. KB has been writing this book her entire life and was honored to partner with her mom and Elizabeth to share her story with others.

www.ingramcontent.com/pod-product-compliance
Lightning Source LLC
Chambersburg PA
CBHW041600260326
41914CB00011B/1329